Essential Oils Allergy Cure:

The Definitive Guide on Using Essential Oils to Completely Eliminate Seasonal Allergy Symptoms

Henry Brooke

Table of Contents

Introduction

I want to thank you for purchasing this book and taking the first step to riding yourself of seasonal allergies naturally. Dealing with allergy symptoms can be a big pain to do. You are going to feel miserable but there is really nothing that you can do about it. You have to continue showing up to work because the symptoms do not warrant going home and medications are not really going to help, so you get to keep trekking through and feeling miserable. This guidebook is going to provide you with a simple solution to dealing with these allergy symptoms so you are able to get back on track: essential oils.

In this book you will learn all about essential oils and how they can help with your allergies. You will learn some of the common symptoms of allergies as well as when things might be serious, how essential oils can help as well as some of their benefits, the best essential oils to use for allergies, and the many different ways to take or apply the oils to get all of their benefits to work for you.

There is just so much that these oils are able to do in order to help you out. Give them a try today and be amazed at how great you can start to feel in no time.

- Henry Brooke

Chapter 1: Common Symptoms of Allergies and Why They Can be a Headache

Dealing with allergies can be a big hassle. They interfere so much with your life but they are not severe enough that you are actually going to be able to get out of the work that you need to get done. Instead, you just have to suffer through them and hope that it all works out for the best and they leave soon.

Many people try to find medications or other remedies that are going to help with the symptoms of their allergies, but often this can make the situation worse because of all the bad side effects or the medication does not work at all. This can just make the whole situation so much more difficult.

Wouldn't it be nice if there were something simple, safe, and effective that you can use in order to get rid of the bad symptoms that come with allergies? Using essential oils is the best way for you to take care of your allergies without having all of the negative things that come with your normal medication. These are all natural so they are going to be safe for your body and can do wonders for making the allergy symptoms go away.

If you are wondering whether you have some of the common symptoms that come with allergies or if it is all in your head, take a look at some of these symptoms before using essential oils to help.

Mild symptoms:

If you are dealing with mild symptoms of allergies, you will notice that you have congestion, itching that is just in one location, and even a rash. The reactions that are considered mild will not go to other body parts.

Moderate symptoms:

In some cases, the symptoms that you have with allergies are going to be a little bit worse. With the mild symptoms, you can sometimes think that you are getting a bit of a cold, but with these they are more defined so you might be able to realize that you have allergies more easily. The symptoms that fall into this category would also be able to spread throughout the body instead of staying in one place.

Some of the symptoms that you may experience with these symptoms include widespread itching all over your body as well as some difficulty in breathing due to inflammation of the breathing tubes.

Severe Symptoms

This is sometimes also called anaphylaxis. Very few people will experience symptoms that are this bad and most of those who do are the ones who are more allergic to food rather than to the pollen outside.

When these symptoms happen, it can often be rare and even life threatening and should be considered as an emergency. It is so critical to the body because the body is reacting to the allergen in such a way that can harm the body and often it is very sudden. It also will affect your whole body rather than just a little area of it which can make the situation turn out even worse for the sufferer.

Sometimes the symptoms are going to start out just mild but they can quickly progress to something that is much more serious. If someone is in contact with a known allergen, they should be rushed to emergency care right away, even if they are not showing any symptoms at that moment.

There are many symptoms that you should look out for when it comes to severe allergy symptoms. These would include:

- Mental confusion and dizziness
- Diarrhea
- Vomiting
- Cramps
- Pain in the stomach
- Swelling—this can be in many different degrees but it is going to make swallowing and breathing very difficult
- Itching face and eyes.

If someone starts to show these symptoms, even if you do not know of an allergy, get them help right away. Failure to get them the help that they need can result in worse issues than if it were handled properly right away.

Confusing with the cold

When it comes to seasonal allergies, many people do not even realize that they are happening. The symptoms that most people undergo, such as the mild ones, are very similar to feeling the common cold. When they strike, people may think that they have the cold rather than the allergies.

Often the best way to tell if you are dealing with seasonal allergies rather than the cold is to look at the time of year. If the seasons are changing, from winter to spring or from summer to fall, and you are going through these symptoms, it is most likely that you have allergies rather than a cold at that time.

Treating allergies with cold medications is not going to do any good for your symptoms. The symptoms will be caused from different sources so the medication for one cannot be translated over to each other. You will have to find special medications to help with the allergies you are dealing with.

The rest of this guidebook will explain how great essential oils can be in helping to alleviate the allergies you are dealing with in a safe and natural way. These are so great and have few, if any, side effects so you will not have to worry about those issues and can work in no time so they really are the best option for your needs.

Chapter 2: Benefits of Using Essential Oils to Help With Allergies

What are Essential Oils

You may be curious to know what essential oils are and how they can be beneficial to your needs. These oils are essentially the liquid that is taken out of plants like aromatic herbs, trees, and flowers.

These oils are able to provide the plant they come from some protection from insects and other things that might bother the plant, but they can also be very effective at keeping you safe and healthy as well.

The essential oil when it is first taken from the plant is going to be very highly concentrated. It also takes a lot of time and effort in order to get some of the oil out of a plant; usually it will take at least one plant and sometimes more to get just one drop of the oil. The wonderful aroma that comes from the oils is the first thing that most people notice about the oils, with the second being how great they are at healing many common health condition.

These oils are very safe and effective since they come naturally from the earth and are not manufactured or combined with other chemicals that can make you sick. This means that you will be able to take the essential oil without worrying about getting harmed. This and the fact that the essential oils are so effective at helping you means that many people are interested in using them to better their lives.

So you may have heard a bit about using essential oils and are wondering if this is a good choice for you. Medications might not have worked for you in the past and you are tired of being stuck with the symptoms that just are not getting better but which are making you feel miserable and you want to try something else.

But you might also be wondering why you should choose to use essential oils? Maybe you have heard some bad things about it in the past and are worried that since many are not regulated that you will get something that is not that good for you. This can often keep some people away from choosing them.

Yes, a few companies might try to fool you, but just reading the directions and ingredients on the package can make it easy to tell if it is a good one for you. Plus there are just so many benefits that come from using essential oils that it would be a shame to miss out on them for your health, especially when it comes to your allergies.

This chapter will talk a bit about some of the many benefits that you are going to get for using essential oils to help with your allergies. You will be surprised at how simple and effective these can be and wonder why you were not brave enough to try out essential oils before now to feel better.

Some of the benefits that you can get form using essential oils include:

1. They can work as antiseptics, anti-infections, anti-parasitic, anti-microbial, antiviral, and anti-fungal. Depending on the type of oil you are using, you

might be able to get several of these benefits from just one. The oils are effective at treating, preventing, and killing off pretty much anything that you have so you can always turn to them to get some help for illnesses.

2. They are good for the body and the mind. You can use some to lift up your spirits and begin to feel better about life. Others are good at aiding your digestion or your heart or even to help you to relax. In the case of the ones listed in the next chapter, they are good at alleviating all of the symptoms that come from allergies so that you can get on with your day.

3. Very powerful antioxidants. This means that they are able to do even more work on your body so that you can be cleared out if there are a lot of toxins or you can keep from getting sick. They are also able to detoxify your cells inside the body so they are able to work more efficiently and give you energy and good health all of the time.

4. They can be used in so many different ways and you can choose to take them in the method that works the best for you. This will be discussed more in the final chapter, but you can choose to take them in pill form, mixed with tea or water, inhaled through a diffusor, used in your cooking, put in a bath, placed on the skin or just smelled straight out of the bottle.

5. They are safe—unlike many of the medications you may be taking, essential oils do not have a lot of chemicals in them that can make you sick. This means that no matter who you are, whether young, old, healthy or not, you will be able to use essential oils for your health.

6. They do not have side effects—the only side effects that you are going to find with the essential oils is that they are helping you to stay in good health. Since these come straight from plants and other things that are found in nature, you are not filling your body up on a lot of bad stuff that can cause it harm, making it the safe choice to use no matter what you need them for.

7. Versatile—all of the essential oils are effective at helping out with at least two different health conditions and some can help with many different health conditions all at the same time. You are not likely to find other medication that is able to do all of this for you so effectively while still remaining safe. The versatility of essential oils also makes them cost effective. You can just get one bottle and use it over and over again, even when allergy season is over, for different purposes so it does not go to waste on you, making it the perfect choice for all of your needs.

8. Help out all parts of your body—not only are you able to get some help with your allergies, you will also find that essential oils are great at helping out every part of your body. Whether you want great looking hair, good breath, faster metabolism, fewer allergies, or happier moods, you will be able to get the help you need from using essential oils.

These are just a few of the benefits that you can get from using essential oils. When it comes to your allergies, they can be really helpful because they are not going to cause harm to your body and will work in a natural way to make the symptoms go away for good. Try out a few of those that are listed below and see just how amazing and efficient that essential oils can be for your body.

Chapter 3: Best Essential Oils for Allergies

When you are ready to begin taking essential oils in order to help out with your seasonal allergies, you are going to want to make sure that you are taking the ones that are going to help you out the best rather than the ones that would work on another health condition. This chapter will explore some of the best essential oils to help out with allergies so that you can start to feel your best.

1. Eucalyptus

Suffering from allergies can be a pain, especially when you are having a lot of trouble breathing and getting in the oxygen that your body needs. This is where this essential oil is going to be able to help you out. You just need to take a bit of this and you will find that your respiratory system is going to open up again because of this essential oils ability to reduce inflammation. So how does this all work?

In a person who does not have allergies, the airways to their lungs are going to be nice and open. The lungs will be able to take in the oxygen with ease back and forth. There will not be any issues to worry about because there is plenty of room for the air to get where it needs to go and all of the parts of the lungs work so that the rest of the body is able to get the oxygen that it needs.

When you are going through an allergy attack, this is not going to continue to happen. Instead of having airways that are nice and wide open for the air to get through, they are going to start closing up and getting smaller. This is because the reactant, or the thing that is causing you to have the allergies such as pollen, is irritating the airways and causing them to go through inflammation. The air has a smaller area to go through and so it feels like it is very painful and difficult to breathe.

When you take the eucalyptus oil, you will find that it is much easier to breathe. This is because the essential oil is effective at reducing the inflammation that you are feeling and instead lets you feel like you can breathe normally. If you are someone who finds that it is really hard to breathe when summer comes along, it is best to give this oil a try.

2. Clove Oil

The next oil that is on our list is clove oil. This one is going to work a little bit differently than the one that was listed above, but it is still going to be able to help you with some of the issues you have concerning allergies.

This essential oil is going to be good as an anti-microbial and an anti-inflammation agent and so it is good at reducing the symptoms of these that come from allergies.

First, it is going to be a good one to work in order to prevent the inflammation that can occur. Instead of taking it like the first one in order to reduce the inflammation that you already have, you will be able to take this one ahead of time, like when you know you will be somewhere that will cause the allergies to flare up, you will be able to take it and be fine.

3. Peppermint

So what all is peppermint able to help you with. It is common that the nasal passages are going to get all stuffed up and smaller when you are dealing with allergies. This means that the nose can feel all stuffed up and like you can't even breathe through it. Even if you are able to breathe through the throat still, it can be really uncomfortable to try and not use your nasal passages like you are used to doing.

Just using a bit of peppermint is the key that you are going to need to use in order to make sure that you are feeling your best all of the time. It is as simple as grabbing a little bottle of essential oil of peppermint and then taking a few sniffs. The concentrated form of peppermint essential oil is strong enough that you will only need to take a few whiffs of the product in order to make yourself feel better. Do not use it for too long because it is so strong that it might start to cause some more irritation to that area than you would like.

4. Lavender

In terms of your allergies, lavender is a good oil to use in order to stop inflammation in the lungs and to reduce the histamine reactions that you are having to the allergies. Not only are you going to need to worry about your body reacting with inflammation when you have allergies, you also have to worry about your histamines being activated and making the issue so much worse. It can cause even more inflammation so that you are having even more troubles with breathing and with the allergies.

When you use the lavender oil, you will be able to avoid both of these problems and so you are able to get on with other things rather than dealing with allergies. How does lavender do this? It is able to help because it is able to calm you down. Often when you are getting upset about the allergies, whether it is because you know the season is around and you are worried about how you react or you are going through a reaction because the allergies are already upon you, you will find that the whole thing is going to become worse. When you take in a bit of lavender, you will find that your body will be able to relax a little bit and feel so much better in the long run.

5. Lemon

Having the smell of lemon oil all around your house can be a great thing. Even if you do not deal with allergies all that much, the lemon is going to make your home smell so much better plus it is a good way to brighten up your mood no matter how sad or down you might be. This all alone is going to make you feel better, but there is so much more that you can do with this oil.

There are a few different ways that lemon oil is going to help you to fight off your allergies. With this lemon oil, you will be able to relieve any of the respiratory issues that you are going through, it can improve your immunity so that you are able to fight off the allergies much better, and then you will also find that it works as an antibacterial and is good at relieving respiratory inflammation.

6. Roman Chamomile

There are many things Roman chamomile is able to help you out with in terms of allergies. We will look at each one in more detail, but basically it helps with easing inflammation that you are feeling, to relieve headaches, to relax, and to be an anti-inflammation.

To start is that it can help with easing the inflammation. If you are already dealing with inflammation because allergy season snuck up on you without any warning, roman chamomile is going to be able to help you out. Also, if you take it ahead of time when you know that you will be outside or in another situation where you might be exposed to the things that cause allergies, you will be able to avoid the inflammation at least a little bit.

When you are dealing with headaches or being stressed out from the allergies, the roman chamomile will help out a lot because it is going to make you calm down and feel so much in the process.

One thing to keep in mind is that you should not use chamomile in order to help with a ragweed allergy. If you are suffering from this, pick another essential oil because the chamomile comes from the same family as the ragweed and is going to make the reaction worse compared to better. There are many other options that you can choose to go with that will work out much better.

7. Frankincense

This is another oil that you might try out if you would like to get relief right away from your stuffy nose or from issues with inflammation in your breathing passages.

Frankincense is also a good choice if you just need to calm down and relax and will work like lavender in helping you out with both of these issues. It is a strong oil that can work wonders for your allergies as well as other parts of your health. The oil that used to be reserved for kings and royalty can now help you to deal with your allergies.

8. Cypress

Cypress is a disinfectant and an antispasmodic. This means that it is going to help keep your body clean of any infections that might come when it has to do with allergies. This can help to keep your immunity strong because it is not fighting off something else when the allergies come to call. When the immune system is nice and strong and it is not worrying about other things, you will be better equipped to deal with the allergies and you might not notice them as much as you did before.

One of the best things that cypress is able to do is to relieve any breathing difficulties that you may be having do to the allergies or from the breathing passages being blocked up. It is also good at suppressing a cough if you happen to get one while you are dealing with the allergies. This is also an essential oils that you should try out when you are suffering from a cold.

9. Ginger

Now you have an excuse to enjoy ginger all of the time or to get the smell of ginger to go all through your home. Ginger is the last essential oil on our list that can be used in order to help you to deal with your allergy symptoms.

This oil is going to work as a stimulant, expectorant, and an analgesic. It is able to decrease the symptoms that you might be feeling in your respiratory system including issues with coughing, wheezing, and constricted breathing. It is also very helpful with any of the upset stomachs or digestive issues that you are having so it is easy to use this oil with any of the other issues that you are dealing with.

Chapter 4: How to Use Essential Oils to Alleviate Allergy Symptoms

Once you have chosen the essential oil that you would like to use for your allergies, you might want to take the time to determine which method you would like to use the essential oil. This chapter will explore some of the most common ways that you can use the oils to get the best results.

Topically

One of the first ways that you can use essential oils in order to deal with your allergy symptoms is to apply it straight to the skin. You can often purchase an ointment of the essential oil and then apply it to your skin or just take it out of the bottle and do it that way. Just remember if you use the essential oil right out of the bottle, make sure to dilute with a carrier oil or else you may cause some irritation to the skin.

One good way to use this topically for allergies is to make a paste of the oil and combine with the carrier oil before placing right on the chest like a Vick's rub. Then you can inhale it in all night and get the great benefits.

Before placing it on the skin, make sure to do a quick test to see if you might have some sensitivity to the oil. To do this, place just a few drops on the underside of your arm, this is the most sensitive part of your body in terms of skin. Leave it there for a few hours to see how you react.

If you see a small rash or feel itchy and irritated, you are probably allergic to the oil and should discontinue use and pick a different kind. There are many that do the same thing so you can choose something else. If after this time you do not see any difference in the skin, the oil is safe to use.

Inhale

Inhaling the essential oil can be just as effective as any of the other methods that will be discussed. Often this is the easiest because you can either do it really quickly or you will be able to just set it up and sit back to relax and enjoy the smell. There are two basic ways to inhale the oil.

First, you can inhale it straight from the bottle. The oil is strong enough to clear up your sinuses and open up the airways to your lungs just by a simple sniff from the bottle. Do this once or twice a day and you are not even using up anything that is in the bottle. Be careful not to do this for the long term or for too long each session; the oil is very concentrated and it can cause irritation to the nose and lungs.

You can also use a diffusor to get the scent of the essential oil into your body. This is a good option if you just want to relax and take in the aroma or if more than one person in the family needs the benefits of the oil. Make sure that you are using a carrier oil with the essential oil or else it is going to be too strong for you to handle. You will also need to stay in the room for a minimum of an hour to get the full benefits from the oil and to get some relief from the allergy symptoms.

In a Bath

Looking for a good way to just relax and let the oils do their job? Taking a bath might be the perfect solution for you. It also has the added benefit of diluting the oil in the water so you do not have to do this part.

In order to take a bath with the oil of your choice and then just add a few drops to the bath water. Let it heat up and fill the bathtub and then just soak and enjoy the delicious feeling that surrounds you while the oil is doing all of the work. You will need to stay in the bath for about 15 minutes, although you can stay in for longer, for the best results before getting out and going on with the day.

In a drink

It is possible to enjoy some essential oil goodness in a nice drink each day. This does not mean that you go out and drink an alcoholic beverage, but you can mix it with pretty much any drink that you want as long as the oil is diluted at least a bit.

This gives you a lot of choices. You can decide to forego the morning coffee and have a nice hot cup of water that is mixed with your essential oil of choice. Add it in to the milk with your cereal to get it done right away. Many people choose to place it in juice because it will mask some of the taste from the oil. It is all up to you what to drink it with, just make sure to get some in each day.

Some essential oils are great to be used in cooking. This is not something that you will be able to do with all of the oils, but there are some that can work well for this. Some might include cloves or even garlic, but others like lavender will not lend themselves all that well to this method of consumption.

When you are doing the cooking method, it is easy to get the oil in. You just add it in as one of the ingredients, in small amounts so that you are not overdoing it, or you can find a recipe that already has the oil in the ingredient list. This is a great method to use because again it allows the whole family to get the benefits of the oil just by eating their dinner and makes it more effective to use.

With all of the methods that you use, it is important that you dilute the oil down a bit, whether it is in your drink, with a carrier oil, in food, or in your bath water. The oil is going to be very strong and can irritate your nose and lungs as well as cause a small rash on the skin or cause some harm to the stomach. Adding in the carrier oil or a method to dilute can prevent these issues and will instead make sure that you are getting the benefits that your body is looking for from the oil.

Conclusion

Thank you for purchasing this book!

I hope this book helps you jumpstart your journey to making seasonal allergies a thing of the past. There are so many things that you can use essential oils for, and your allergies can feel the amazing effects in no time. Try out a few of the oils that are listed in this guidebook as well as some of the tips in order to get started with relieving your allergy symptoms in no time!

Finally, if you enjoyed this book, then I'd like to ask you for a favor, would you be kind enough to leave a review for this book on Amazon? It'd be greatly appreciated!

Thank you and good luck!

- Henry Brooke

Ashley Fitzgerald

SEX: THE SERIAL ORGASMIC WOMAN
When Just One is not Enough

© 2015 by Michael Winicott.

© 2015 by UNITEXTO

Published by UNITEXTO

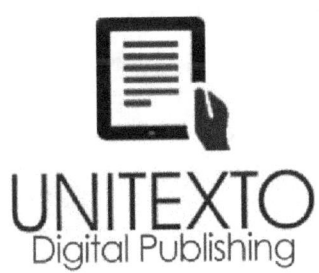

UNITEXTO
Digital Publishing